PRESCHOOL

PLUGGED-IN PLANNER

WRITTEN BY

Screen Sanity

IN PARTNERSHIP WITH SUSAN CROWN EXCHANGE

To order additional copies of this resource visit **screensanity.org/tools** or email at **info@screensanity.org.**

SO GLAD
YOU'RE HERE.

Welcome!

Before you dive in, please take a moment to give yourself a pat on the back — you picked up this planner and are taking action. Kudos to you! Raising kids in today's increasingly digital world is not an easy task. Our children will never know a world without smartphones and social media, having a completely different experience than we did. On top of that, today's parents feel pressure from countless outside influences (social media, doctors, grandparents, work, news reports, etc.) and it's easy to feel overwhelmed and lost.

We're here to let you know you're not alone. We get it. And please remember: there's no perfect way to embark on this journey. There will certainly be hiccups along the road. However, it's never too early to start preparing your family for the digital world.

Our hope is this planner helps you look ahead and proactively consider the role technology plays in your child's earliest years. Together, we can create a world where kids are **captivated by life, not screens.**

CONSIDER THE BIG PICTURE

When it comes to device introduction, three words guide our process: **"Ride. Practice. Drive."** Teaching your kid to drive a device is sort of like teaching your kid to drive a car. Similar to driver's ed, there can be an intentional process to introducing new technology.

In navigating this roadmap, it may be helpful to identify where your child is on their digital journey. Take some time to orient yourself on the following map, envisioning what your child's device use will entail in the coming years.

This will look different for every family. The end goal is not to find the magic age or correct plan, but rather to familiarize yourself with the path you plan/hope to take.

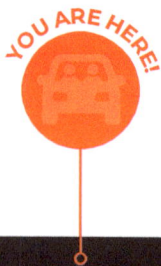

YOU ARE HERE!

| RIDE | PRACTICE | DRIVE |

This planner is focused on supporting parents with kids in the in the early stages of device introduction.

RIDE

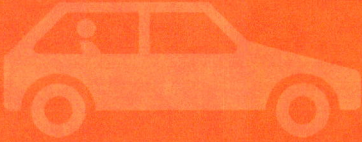

Buckle up in the back.
Start by having your child observe your digital practices and device use, similar to how we watched our parents drive from the backseat.

PRACTICE

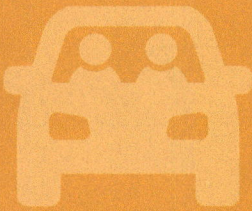

Start small.
When it's time for a device, consider one that is simple, safe and stripped down to limited features. Allow your kid to experiment with independence and develop foundational skills. During this time, plan to log many hours riding in the passenger seat, helping them practice healthy digital habits.

DRIVE

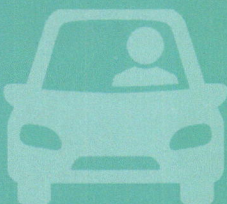

Smartphone independence.
When he or she demonstrates competence and you feel comfortable, your child is likely ready to embark on solo device use. They'll still bump curbs or get into accidents, but they can mostly navigate sticky situations on their own.

1/

THEN + NOW

Today, technology greets our children from the time they're born, making it nearly impossible to avoid the world of screens. Unlike the snail-mail baby announcements of yesteryear, a new baby's arrival is often proudly posted on social media within hours of its arrival — that is, if Grandma didn't get to it first!

Smartphones allow us to capture these precious early moments and help us introduce new arrivals to eager family members via video-calls. Yet, our children's interaction with screens is not always so straightforward.

While we'd love to give you specifics on the perfect age for device introduction or the magic number of screentime minutes, the truth is every family (and every child) is different.

What we can say is that there are ways to be intentional and equipped when introducing your kids to devices and the online world. Let's start by looking back at your own experiences with technology.

Remember Your Inner Child

Describe a memory from your childhood when you shared time on screens with someone you loved. Maybe a movie you saw in theaters or a TV show you used to watch together?

_____

_____

What made the above experience enjoyable? Can that feeling or experience be recreated with your child today?

_____

_____

Remember what you want to recreate from your childhood and envision your child's relationship with screens over the next couple years. What values will you keep in mind to guide you in structuring their time in the digital world?

☐ Community	☐ Faith	☐ Integrity	☐ Service
☐ Connection	☐ Friendship	☐ Kindness	☐ Sustainability
☐ Creativity	☐ Giving	☐ Love	☐ Teamwork
☐ Determination	☐ Grace	☐ Productivity	☐ Tolerance
☐ Empathy	☐ Gratitude	☐ Recreation	☐ Trust
☐ Encouragement	☐ Hard Work	☐ Respect	☐ _____
☐ Exploration	☐ Honor	☐ Self-Improvement	☐ _____

What side effects of screens do you want to avoid? What worries you most about introducing technology to your child?

_____

_____

Recreate the Magic

Time to dream cast! **Create a bucket list of experiences** you hope to share with your child, screen-related and beyond — moments to experience, shows to watch, laughs to share. There are obstacle courses to be built and car playlists to be made. Childhood can be full of pretend tea parties and sock-puppet plays if we make time to fully engage. Take some inspiration from the beloved Australian cartoon _Bluey_. In this clever (often tear-inducing) series, Bluey and her family share countless off-screen adventures, putting a spotlight on the importance of fostering childhood wonder and joining in imaginative play.

CONNECTION AS A CORE VALUE

The Still Face Experiment, originally conducted in 1975 and replicated numerous times since, powerfully illustrates the necessity of connection for our youngest ones.

Developmental psychologist Edward Tronick's findings show that when infants meet a nonresponsive, expressionless parent, it takes only three minutes before they grow wary, withdraw and exhibit a look of hopelessness.

Connection — even in infancy — is one of the most important aspects of the human experience.

▷|◁ **REFLECT**

Disconnect to Connect

Take a moment to reflect on your bond and connection with your child.

What activities or routines make you feel most connected to your child?

☐ Building forts   ☐ Cooking   ☐ Dance parties
☐ Dressing up   ☐ Exploring outside   ☐ Going to the playground
☐ Making crafts   ☐ Playing make-believe   ☐ _____
☐ Reading   ☐ Singing   ☐ _____

How do you show your child love? How does he or she show you love?

_____
_____

Identify times you notice technology (phones, tablets, TVs, etc.) **disrupting** your connection with your child.

_____
_____

Identify times you notice technology (phones, tablets, TVs, etc.) **enhancing** your connection with your child.

_____
_____

⚡ **PLUG IN**

Provide a Looking Glass

When we were younger, we watched our parents pay bills on paper, shop for groceries in person, read printed newspapers or call to make doctor appointments. Today, we can conveniently complete these adult tasks on our devices. Yet, we often forget that what our children observe is a device winning our attention over them. Next time you're using your phone for household tasks, try narrating what you're doing. This not only signals to our kids that we aren't ignoring them, it also helps them understand that screens can be beautiful tools for connection and productivity.

This could sound something like:

"Hey Jack, I'm putting in a grocery order on my phone right now. What snacks would you like me to add? Can you help me look for something?"

3/

STARTING WITH YOURSELF

You are your child's biggest role model at this early stage in their life. Kids notice everything about your daily routines, from where you put your shoes to how you sip your cup of morning coffee — device-use included.

As they get older, they'll start paying attention to things you share on Instagram and pin on Pinterest. Your habits reveal what types of things you value and celebrate, and what things you don't.

Now, hold the panic — this doesn't mean you have to have perfect screen habits (here's a secret: they don't exist). It just means being aware of what beliefs your kiddo internalizes, and cognizant of times when you might be fading into the background, distracted by your screen, rather than remaining present in the memory-making. Give yourself grace and compassion as you reflect honestly on your relationship with screens.

Recognize Habits

How do you feel about your relationship with your phone?

Got things under control ①—②—③—④—⑤—⑥—⑦—⑧—⑨—⑩ Totally overwhelmed

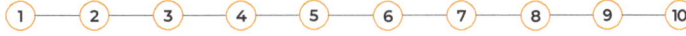

Describe a time when your child imitated something about your tech use. How did that make you feel?

_____

_____

_____

Set Intentions

There is no magic wand when it comes to finding the right screen-life balance, but small tweaks can make a world of difference in your digital health. **Check one or two steps you would like to take:**

☐ **Turn off notifications.**
Unless they're from a real person (like texts or calls) it can be helpful to eliminate those tempting little dings.

☐ **Wear a smartwatch to filter out notifications.**
This helpful trick can allow you to be "on call" to the few people who need to get through to you — spouses, caregivers and the school nurse — while allowing your phone to stay in your pocket.

☐ **Give your phone a spring cleaning.**
Give yourself permission to get rid of things that don't spark joy. The app that steals time and attention? Try deleting it (or moving it off your home page). That person on Instagram that makes you feel bad? It's okay to unfollow them.

☐ **Apply friction.**
Consider inserting tiny obstacles that make it a little harder to mindlessly reach for your screen. Get creative about ways you can disrupt bad screen habits and adopt healthier ones.
- ○ Keep your phone in a desk drawer when working
- ○ Use a device other than your phone for an alarm clock
- ○ Charge devices outside of your bedroom
- ○ Remove distracting apps from your homescreen
- ○ Adjust screentime limit settings

DEVICE-FREE ZONES

While our little ones often reach for devices, deep down, they also dream about quality screen-free time.

In 2017, the city of Boston asked all kindergarteners to design the best playground imaginable. Like the planners, you may envision twisty slides, splash pads and sand pits.

But, to their surprise, the overwhelming top request from the kindergarteners was nothing of the sort. The main thing the kids were after? **Playgrounds that required lockers for their parents to put away their phones.**

Kids would rather pretend the floor is lava — jumping from pillow to pillow — than play on a tablet; they just need our help establishing device-free zones.

If you're looking for a good place to start, we suggest tables and bedtimes.

▷|◁ **REFLECT**

Set Your Boundaries

When are times in the day where you have the opportunity for meaningful connection with your child?

_____

_____

What are times and spaces where you hope to create device-free zones:

- ☐ Bedrooms
- ☐ Bathrooms
- ☐ During meals
- ☐ Vacations
- ☐ In the car
  (except on long trips)

- ☐ With babysitters/caregivers
- ☐ Pool/playground
- ☐ During playdates/playgroups
- ☐ During classes/activities
- ☐ _____
- ☐ _____

One of the healthiest things you can do for your child is set a norm that devices aren't in their bedroom at night. This can protect their valuable sleep. If you're interested in doing this, consider the following:

Where will they charge?

☐ Kitchen   ☐ Home Office   ☐ Parent's room   ☐ _____

Tip: When putting devices to sleep it can help to utlize a timer or adjust the device settings to apply limits or downtime.

⚡ **PLUG IN**

Device-Free Outings

The next time you go to a park playdate or story time at the library, consider making it a device-free outing. Your child might not have their own phone yet, but by setting an expectation now, you'll create a template for later, when it's time for them to start putting their own device down. The secret sauce to making it stick? **Use a catchy phrase, such as "phone away, it's time to play" or "phone time ends when we're with our friends."**

Feel free to get creative and make your own! Exercising this muscle now — by demonstrating how you put your device away — will soften larger battles down the road. It would be neat if we all had an inner voice that said, "When I'm with people or when I need to focus, my phone doesn't get to join."

5 /

WEAR YOUR SEATBELT

We all want to keep our kids safe in the **real world.** We remind them to buckle up when getting in the car, look both ways before crossing the street, be cautious around a campfire and wash hands before meals. In the same way, we need to prepare our kids for the hazards of the **digital world,** where predators, cyberbullies and pornbots abound.

Shockingly, the average age of first porn exposure is just nine years old. Young eyes are often exposed to more mature content than we are aware, so it's never too early to safeguard your child's online environment. Think of these precautions like a seatbelt — offering your child as much protection as possible from accidents in the online world.

▷|◁ **REFLECT**

Safety First

While no solution is 100% foolproof, there are many safety nets you can put in place. Which will you use for your child?

☐ **Apply filters on home routers/Wi-fi** to help to keep hardcore content out of your child's digital experience.

☐ **Avoid allowing use of devices in private** to observe your child during time on screens. Keeping headphones unplugged can also allow you to keep an ear out for anything that may flag your concern.

☐ **Turn off location on devices** to provide privacy and prevent location tracking.

How will you prepare your child to respond when violent or inappropriate content appears on their screen?

☐ Look away
☐ Close the device like Pacman

☐ Toggle to home screen
☐ Let a trusted adult know

Even with safety nets in place, mistakes happen. When your child shares — or you uncover — an awkward or shocking situation, it's critical you don't overreact. Pick a phrase you want to practice to help you keep your "poker face."

☐ Tell me more.
☐ Thanks so much for trusting me with this.
☐ Gosh, that's interesting. How did that make you feel?

☐ I'd love to hear more. Want to grab some ice cream?
☐ I'm so glad you know you can tell me anything.

Pick a code word you can establish with your kids so they feel equipped when they see something inappropriate and need to talk:

_____

⚡ **PLUG IN**

Be Proactive

We know starting a conversation about hazards like pornography is easier said than done — but there is hope. We recommend reading the book *Good Pictures Bad Pictures Jr.* with your child. This internationally acclaimed, read-aloud book empowers younger children with the Turn, Run & Tell plan for keeping safe online. We found it to be gentle and effective in introducing conversations about the topic in a comfortable, compelling way.

RHYTHMS ARE YOUR FRIEND

As you know, the terrible twos are unfortunately not a myth or old wives' tale. Leaving a toy behind or switching to a new snack is no big deal — until it is.

And devices can sometimes cause the worst tantrums of all. In national surveys, parents share that the number one battleground in their homes is technology. So how can we defuse tension without throwing in the towel? **Consider creating steady routines and screentime habits.**

Establishing healthy rhythms is not for the faint of heart. This is tough work, especially at the beginning. But, soon enough, when consistency is held, the predicable patterns will take the fall for being the bad guy and you will be let off the hook. Forming rhythms now will help you fight less battles in the long run.

Write Your Rhythm

Take a moment and brainstorm a technology rhythm that can become your family's mantra. Don't stress about how other families do it — just create something attainable, that supports your family's unique needs. Here are a couple of examples to use as inspiration:

(1) Less screentime, more dreamtime.

(2) No screens before noon.

(3) Tablet up. Teeth brushed. Books read. Time for bed.

(4) Set the tech timer.

Consider striving for a 1:1 online to offline ratio. For every half hour spent engaged with screens, we encourage a half hour spent engaged with real life. Or maybe you call this your Rule of 30: For every 30 minutes of time with tech, you have 30 minutes of unplugged time.

Feeling inspired? Create your own:

_____

_____

⚡ **PLUG IN**

Plan Together

Include your kids in this conversation. Having ownership over new routines can help reduce the battle. If kids have a choice between different rhythms, or to be a part of the creation, they'll be less likely to resist.

Perhaps you schedule a time during the week, at dinner or over breakfast, to plan out your offline activities for the upcoming weekend. Does your child want to go to the zoo or on a hike? Try a new restaurant every Friday? Schedule Saturday as movie night? Make a list of activities that become routine. You might be surprised by how the ideas your kids add become family traditions.

AVOIDING MELTDOWNS

Our brains naturally adapt to their environment, however the world of screens and the real world run at distinctly different paces.

When our kids are asked to "hop off" screens, the experience can be like the moment you step off a merry-go-round. Their brains are sped up and out of sync with the pace of the world. As you're likely aware, this mismatch can sometimes present itself in loud and ugly ways.

Your challenge — should you choose to accept it — is to **help them log off before their brains have reached the point of no return**...and then help them sync back up with the world around them.

See the Change

The number one indicator that your child's brain has reached its limit is behavior change. When you notice this happening, it's a sign they'll need your help in co-regulating their emotions and decision-making.

When and where do you find it most difficult to transition off screens without a meltdown? Can you identify "early indicators" that a meltdown is coming?

Meltdown Indicators

☐ Agression   ☐ Exhaustion   ☐ Refusing choices

☐ Repetitive movements   ☐ Shouting   ☐ _____

What are some things you might try to help your child learn to transition off screens without a meltdown?

☐ Touch them on the shoulder

☐ Use calm language like, "Find a good place to stop."

☐ Set a timer to display screentime minutes

☐ Allow them to finish the activity they have been working on

☐ Engage them in an activity when they log off

☐ Narrate your own transitions out loud to model a healthy approach

What activities best help your child reset after they log off?

☐ Going outside   ☐ Building with playdough

☐ Helping prep dinner   ☐ Free play time

☐ Performing household chores   ☐ Reading books

☐ Coloring or painting   ☐ _____

Think Ahead

While screens can be the cause of many meltdowns, it's also often used as an easy cure. **The temptation to hand your child a phone during a tantrum is all too real.** Yet, if we make a habit of this, our kids lose opportunities to develop crucial self-coping and emotional regulation skills. To be prepared in those moments when the voice in the back of your head is saying, "maybe this isn't such a good idea, but it's convenient," consider throwing an activity or game in your bag or car. Maybe you can even try to involve your kiddo in the shopping experience. Can you make a game of "I spy" in the aisles or have them count the items in the cart? There may still be days when our creative muscles are tired and we turn to screens as the solution, but thinking ahead with a plan can reduce the frequency.

QUALITY VS. QUANTITY

The digital world wants to keep you scrolling, but at the end of life, all you have is your time and attention.

When you look back, what will you (and your child) say was time well spent?

What if instead of a platform for endless consumption, screens were intentionally used to spark creation?

One of the most forward-thinking things we can do as parents is to team up with technology, helping our kids see it as a means to an end — a mode for driving creativity, curiosity and connection — and not the goal itself.

▷|◁ REFLECT

Plugged With Purpose

What are ways your child enjoys being creative or things your child likes to create? Are they an expert in playdough pizzas, a fashion connoisseur or a shadow puppet extraordinaire? Do they put on dance performances or build elaborate LEGO formations? How do they enjoy engaging with the world around them?

_____

_____

At Screen Sanity, we often divide our interactions with technology into three categories: creation, consumption and connection. What are some ways your child's screen use falls into each of the following? We've started you off with a few ideas.

Creation

☐ Draw along videos
☐ Making new recipes
☐ Creating finger puppets
☐ _____

Connection

☐ Video calls with family
☐ Watch a show together
☐ Storytime hour
☐ _____

Consumption

☐ Watching movies/videos
☐ Educational apps/games
☐ Listening to music
☐ _____

Are there factors that lead your child's tech use to fall more into a certain category? How can you tip the scale to protect time well spent?

_____

_____

PLUG IN

Capture Creativity

Take a moment to reflect on how you liked to play as a child and see if you can **recapture that creativity in your digital world.** Maybe this is researching and reading about something that piques your curiosity, something you never have time to sit down and learn about. Or, maybe it's using your social media as a creative writing outlet instead of a scroll-fest. Once you experiment with this concept, invite your kiddo to join you in engaging with technology in a higher quality way. Look up simple crafts to create, learn words in sign language or help them research their favorite animal. The possibilities are endless, and the fun has just begun!

For more ideas, download our **30 Days of Creation PDF** _at screensanity.org._

9 /

FIND YOUR PEOPLE

Raising kids in this digital world is hard, but it's even harder to do it alone. Similar to when our kids start eating solid foods or begin the potty-training journey, it's helpful to link arms regarding tech use. It can be overwhelming to start a conversation about screens with other parents, but the sooner you start, the more you will benefit and "get ahead" of the challenges to come.

⊳|⊲ **REFLECT**

Start a Convo

Is there someone you feel safe talking to as you navigate the challenges of raising kids in a digital world?

_____

_____

Is there someone you need to communicate your tech boundaries or concerns with? What are your hesitations — and what is the best possible outcome?

_____

_____

Tip: Our **Babysitter Guide** _is a helpful tool for easily sharing important information with your caregivers, including phone numbers, activity ideas and your family's unique tech boundaries. Visit screensanity.org to download._

⚡ **PLUG IN**

Link Arms

As parents, we share everything from favorite snacks to the best go-to babysitters. When it comes to screentime, starting a Screen Sanity Group Study or hosting a Screen Sanity Parent Night can be a great way to create a safe, non-judgmental space to answer the questions we're all pondering.

This can look like gathering around a kitchen table with your book club, or joining your PTA in the local library, or even inviting your neighbors to gather in the backyard as the kids blow bubbles and play in the sprinkler. Visit our website at **screensanity.org** for more info on starting a group or hosting a parent night.

You were never meant to do life alone, so let's continue this journey together!

Screen Sanity is here for you at each milestone and tech-related challenge.

Continue to stay "plugged in" with our next two books,

the Elementary School Plugged-in Planner and the Middle School Plugged-in Planner.

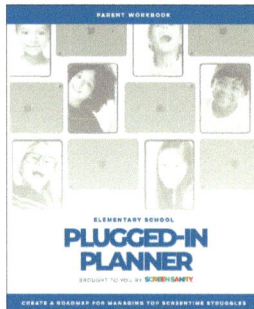

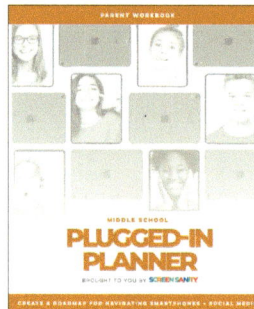

SCREENSANITY.ORG

Notes

www.ingramcontent.com/pod-product-compliance
Lightning Source LLC
Chambersburg PA
CBHW041106050426
42335CB00047B/173

*9 7 9 8 9 8 7 3 0 8 4 1 7 *